THE FAT GIRL
CHRONICLES

THE FAT GIRL CHRONICLES

◆

A HANDBOOK FOR FAT CHICKS

THE LIFE STORY AND SITUATION ABOUT BEING FAT AND LEARNING TO ACCEPT MYSELF

Kimberly M. Denesse

iUniverse, Inc.
New York Lincoln Shanghai

THE FAT GIRL CHRONICLES
A HANDBOOK FOR FAT CHICKS

Copyright © 2006 by Kimberly M Denesse

iUniverse books may be ordered through booksellers or by contacting:

iUniverse
2021 Pine Lake Road, Suite 100
Lincoln, NE 68512
www.iuniverse.com
1-800-Authors (1-800-288-4677)

ISBN-13: 978-0-595-38391-7 (pbk)
ISBN-13: 978-0-595-82764-0 (ebk)
ISBN-10: 0-595-38391-2 (pbk)
ISBN-10: 0-595-82764-0 (ebk)

Printed in the United States of America

THANK YOU

TO MY MOTHER AND FATHER,
MY CHILDREN,
MY FRIENDS FOR BEING THERE

TO THOSE WHO DIDN'T ACCEPT ME FOR WHO I AM,
THANK YOU
FOR MAKING ME STRONG

TO MW FOR GETTING ME TO LAUGH AT MYSELF

TO MY ENTIRE FAMILY FOR BEING WHO YOU ARE

AND TO GOD FOR BLESSING ME AND KEEPING ME IN HIS
GRACES

Foreward

When the idea for this handbook came to me, I had no idea how to write it. I wasn't sure where to begin let alone end the story that would have so much of myself in it. Then I decided to just-begin. That's the best way to put it.

Some will think it odd of me to want to write something like this but I feel as though it needed to be done. I have grown tired of always being exposed to a world where the only way people are happy is if they are thin. That's not my dream in life nor is it the key to my happiness and I am certain there are others who feel the same way.

I remember times where my mother would say to me "Do you know why you are so unhappy all the time? It's because you're so fat. Lose weight and you'll be happier."
For a while, I believed her. Until I realized that my unhappiness was due to the fact that I was letting others make me feel uncomfortable about being fat.
I never noticed it because I was always trying to make others happy instead of focusing on myself and what made me happy and satisfied. But, when I finally made that connection, I began to heal.

Now, don't get me wrong, I'm not saying that people shouldn't exercise and eat healthier. I'm just saying that you can't always equate being thin with being happy nor can you always equate being fat with depression. Besides, there's nothing wrong with being happy and satisfied just the way you are. That's the point of the handbook. I want everyone who reads it to make a decision to love themselves on THEIR TERMS. Not someone else's.

I'm not expecting to make lots of money or even become incredibly popular. I just want to spread the message that loving yourself is what's important. I think many of us forget that point in the hustle and bustle of everyday life trying to keep things focused and going right in this day and age.

So, I hope whomever decides to pick this book up and thumb through the pages, or maybe even buy it, enjoys it. I hope it gives you the ability to laugh, maybe even cry. But, most importantly, I want it to make you realize that you shouldn't try to conform to what others want you to be.

Pleasant reading to all…

~Kimberly M. Denesse

THE CURVE OF HER FACE,
THE WARMTH OF THAT PLACE

GENTLE HILLS,
NO SPACE IS CONCEALED
THE PASSION THAT FILLS
HER WOMANHOOD REVEALED

THE MYSTERIES THAT MESMERIZE,
FEELINGS FLOW FREELY,
THE WARMTH OF HER THIGHS,
THE IDEA OF THIS IMPOSSIBILITY

THE SOFTNESS OF HER SKIN,
A SMELL OF SWEETNESS,
HER TRUE BEAUTY HELD WITHIN.

FAT: MORE THAN JUST A WORD

Many people will wonder why I have chosen to write a book such as this one.

Many will wonder why I have chosen to expose my deepest, darkest feelings about being fat to the world. Well, I'm not even sure if that is a question that I can easily answer. So many reasons come to mind for me to state here on these pages, but I'm not even sure if anyone would even understand them. One thing I know for certain is that it is something that needs to be done. I guess I can just say that I am tired of people's perceptions of fat people: fat, hopeless, lonely and disgusting.

Yes. Disgusting.

I'm only saying what thousands, millions of people think about us fat folks everyday. I'm just getting sick of seeing us portrayed as the fat, lazy, lonely slobs in movies and on television.

You know what I'm talking about.

The fat girl that all the guys poke fun of and run away from.

The dirty fat guy that repulses all the ladies.

Those images have long been looked at as what most fat folks are and I'm here to make a strong objection to it.

What?

Are you shocked that I'm using the word fat?

Fatfatfafatfatfatfatfatfatfatfat.

Fat.

Does it make you uncomfortable?

Whether you're fat or not, it makes people ill at ease to hear it. Like it's some kind of voodoo curse.

Give me a damn break.

It is just a word.

Get over it already.

I just want to show everyone that we are people with feelings and problems just like the perfect beauties you see everyday on television. It's just that fat people are less appealing than "normal" folks and that makes us an easy target for the world to point and laugh at; to tease with terrible words.

And to feel pity because they think we are weak.

But, we have faces, lives, and feelings.

I'm writing this to show everyone that just because I'm fat, doesn't mean I'm not worthy of respect or love.

IN THE BEGINING

To put it plainly, I am a person who has struggled with weight issues for the better part of my short life. I was always the biggest kid in dance class. My mother would joke because she said in order to find me on stage, all she had to do was look for the chunky thighs. I was made fun of in elementary school, junior high and sometimes I was even teased in high school for being heavy. After the birth of my second son, my weight became a serious, serious issue for me. You know what happened? I let myself get fat.

Yes.

I let it happen.

There is no other reason or explanation other than the fact that I did nothing about gaining weight.

No medical reason.
No family history.
It's just that plain and simple.

Now, don't get me wrong. I'm not saying that it's everyone's reason for getting fat. Some people do have family history or medical issues to take into account. I'm just saying that I, like many others, just turned a blind eye to the weight gain. My emotions had much to do with it.

I'm an emotional eater.

Just like plenty of people out there.

It doesn't make me weak. It's just the thing I use to smother my fears, my pain, and my anger. It is my drug of choice. Some people use drugs or alcohol to hide behind their pain. But, we are all the same in the respect that we pick some unhealthy habit to hide behind. Does that make the beauty queen who abuses prescription drugs any better than me? Or the athlete who uses cocaine?

No.

We are all the same. It's just that my addiction shows itself in a way that it is displayed for all the world to see.

Food has always been at the center of my life. So, it was easy for me to get addicted to it. I live in a city where people "live to eat" rather than eating to live. So, you can imagine how easy it is to get your hands on any and everything a food addict could possibly want. Especially at home and in my family life.

We plan holidays, parties, celebrations and the first thing to discuss is food. It doesn't help that members on both sides of my family happen to be wonderful cooks. So, I've got it shooting right at me with both barrels loaded.

I don't really recall the exact moment I began to overeat. (Or eat whenever my emotions were out of control). But, to get to the root cause of my overeating and my basic addiction to food, I need to delve deeper into my twisted mind to figure out at which point did it go from "enjoying" to "dependency" on food.

I do know that there are many moments in my life when I went back to the pot to fill my plate over and over and over again. Or times when I hid food to hoard it like I was a starving child. The impulse to overeat was so strong I couldn't control it. I would eat peanut butter and jelly out of a coffee mug. I would hide food under my bed to eat at night after everyone else had gone to sleep. I would go to the store and buy junk food and eat it until it was all gone and there was nothing left. I would eat and eat until there was nothing left. I would eat until I got sick.

It's like feeding some horrible monster that you can't see or hear. But you feel it gnawing at your insides. Consuming every bit of you. And every day it gets more and more out of control. No one else sees it, but you know it's there and you're forced to deal with its hideous power all by yourself.

I suppose that is what makes it so easy for family, friends and strangers to tease or put a fat person down because they think you're just eating because you're greedy. They don't know that sometimes it's something much more horrible going on inside. I guess if our addictions were to actual drugs then they would be concerned with trying to find out what types of emotional issues we were having. But it's always easier to just look on in disgust and call you a fat pig rather than ask if you're feeling ok.

I know how that feels. I was on the receiving end of more than one pointed finger telling me how disgusting I was. But, I realize that even if they hadn't said those words, even if they had just said that my eating habits were unhealthy, I would've eaten myself into oblivion anyway. That's just how it is. I was hiding from all of the things that terrified me. I was hiding away from the terrible things that happened to me. I was hiding from the world. Food was my way of covering up, of ignoring all of the things that would force themselves to the surface. But in the end, the only thing I ended up hiding from was **ME**. I covered myself up in this layer of shame, fear, guilt, and sorrow instead of facing my pain, my fear. I turned around and let it destroy almost every piece of the real me.

One day, I just looked at myself and thought "Don't do this anymore"

And that is how my recovery began. This book is part of that recovery.

I know to many people, the way I talk about eating and hiding food, they will find it disgusting. But, there are those out there who do the same thing I did. They know what it's like and I am exposing myself on their behalf. I want them to know that they are not alone. I also want them to know that at some point, you need to break the cycle. Stop feeding those demons that linger on the inside. Face them and let them go. It's a long process and I am still learning although I have come a long a way. It's never easy to open up and expose everything that hides within you. It's never easy when you have to face yourself.

Your **_REAL_** self that hides beneath the layers and behind the Oreo cookies.

The process for me, has not been simple. Nor will it ever be. It's never easy when you struggle with addictions to food everyday of your life. But, it's a process; it constantly changes and evolves until something better is made.

One thing I want to stress to everyone reading these pages is that just because you're fat, there is nothing for you to be ashamed of, nothing to hate yourself for and no reason to think that you are the only person going through these things.

We are fragile, imperfect and strange at times. We don't like to face the unpleasantries of life in any form or manner. We barely like to face ourselves in the mirror sometimes. But, that is how it goes. And whether we develop addictions to certain things or people, it should not be something that shames us. You learn to let go of that dependency and you grow as a person. My biggest fear in life is not being accepted. Your biggest fear in life is not being accepted. Everyone's fear in life is not being accepted. But the biggest part to that all is that one should accept them first and foremost. Damn if the next guy does or not.

That is another aspect of food: It accepts you just the way you are. It doesn't talk or hit or insult you. It just is. And even though I am learning to let go of these "food demons" that I have, one thing remains: *I am still a fat girl*. Whether other people like it or not, that is me. It is a matter of letting go of the unacceptable and accepting the imperfection. Besides, overeating isn't the only hazard of the trade. Binge and purge or starving yourself is another unfortunate side of things. It is a sad thing to know that people are so afraid of being fat. I mean, don't get me wrong, it's not an easy situation to handle. But, it in no way means that you are doomed forever to some horrible existence just because you are fat. We all search for acceptance in so many ways, with other people, instead of with ourselves. WE make ourselves unacceptable. No matter what our appearance may be, WE are always unhappy with the way we look. We search for ways to make ourselves look better, to be more appealing to everyone else. What about being appealing to us? That seems to be something that is always overlooked. We search for so much, in the wrong places. What about within ourselves. In our hearts, for what will truly make us happy. You can diet and take pills; even get surgery, but does it really solve the problem for everyone? I am not knocking these options. Trust me, I have either tried or contemplated many solutions to my own weight problem. I am not knocking the fact that many people are really happy after they have lost weight. But is it the thing for everyone. That is the issue. I have come to face the fact that my issues with food and my weight are not just going to be easily solved by repairing it with some false overlay. I have come to see that the issue must be worked on from the inside out FIRST.

So, how do you come to face the **REAL** issues with yourself? Well, you start by looking in the mirror. Face that person you have been hiding from for all of those years and be completely, totally and yes, brutally honest with them.

Ask yourself, "face-to-face", what is it that we have hated about ourselves for all of these years?

Why do we continue to damage our self-esteem?

And finally, is it more important for Society to accept us or more important that we learn to accept ourselves?

On my personal journey, I had to ask myself these questions and I also had to keep reminding myself that I have to live with me and that whatever damage I do, I am the one that has to deal with it. I have chosen to start facing facts and dealing with the reality that it is completely and totally unrealistic of me to think that I will ever look like swimsuit-modelvideochick. It is also unrealistic of me to think that I will only be happy if I finally looked like swimsuitmodelvideochic. Although I am quite certain that life would certainly be much, MUCH easier for me if I looked like that. I could probably find better fitting clothes, cheaper clothes, and I could probably find some really hot, sexy, shallow guy that only wants me for my body.

HAHA.

I just thought I'd throw that in. Just to see if you're paying attention. Not all guys are shallow, so please forgive me for that one.

But let's move on...Shall we?

When you look at me, what is it that you see?
Do you see that which is truly me?

Finding beauty in my brain,
Even though I am simple and plain

Choosing me because I'm really smart,
Wanting to know what lies deep in my heart

Seeing beyond the outside,
To see the beautiful woman that exists on the inside

When you look at me, what is it, honestly, that you truly see?
Do you see what is the false side of me?

Falling in love with the outside,
Ignoring the selfishness that I don't even try to hide

Using you and you don't seem to care,
Only seeing me for all the skin that I bear

Nothing but fakeness in my heart,
But you don't care that I'm not smart

As long as I impress your family and friends,
You don't care if this lie never ends

You never look at the real me,
Choosing only to see
The wrong things,
Never the good things

Me
Me

You never see the real me,
Choosing only to see,

The false side,
The wrong side of me.

Look
Look
At me.
For me.
The real me.

WHOSE IDEA WAS IT ANYWAY?

I know that my problems are emotional. I know that I am fat because I overeat at times. But, I'm not depressed because I'm fat. I'm depressed because of emotional problems. There's a difference.

People always want to put being fat at the top of the "That's why you're depressed list". It's not that way for everyone. I certainly wish that the folks who come up with the ideas for weight loss commercials get that point as well.

Have you seen some of them lately?

They disgust me.
How dare they try to portray fat people as lonely and unhappy.

The Jenny Craig commercial has Kirstie Alley walking down the street, surrounded by men leering and howling at her. One guy says "She looks great" and Kirstie turns around and says "Is he talking to me??"
She has this look of surprise and rips off her coat and suddenly she's surrounded by men and they are all dancing in the street.

Guess what's playing?
"It's Raining Men".
Then the announcer comes over and starts saying how much weight Kirstie lost and join Jenny Craig blah blah blah.

I was pissed when I saw it.

How dare they.
Don't think that just because I'm fat I don't get guys looking at me or that I don't get dates or anything of the sort.

I knew that eventually it would come down to them (advertisers) playing on insecurities and emotions to get people to spend money and join their program.

I think it's great that Kirstie Alley is happy now that she's dropped some weight. But don't imply that fat women are lonely and can't get guys without losing weight.

The other commercial is Weight Watchers.
Now, I've joined their program several times. But, I realize that I only did it because someone else urged me to join. So, the program never worked and I only went a few times.

That commercial consists of them showing different women in different situations. One is at a party feeling like "the fattest woman in the room". Another is feeling lonely, watching everyone else on dates having a good time.
The song playing is Chers' "This is a song for the lonely".

Oh yeah, this one really makes me want to wretch.

They show the ladies at the end, joining Weight Watchers, losing weight and suddenly they aren't lonely nor are they the fattest women in the room.

Hooray for anyone that losses weight and feels better because of it. But why is it the fat woman that's always lonely or uncomfortable? Why is it the fat woman that's always without a date?

I hatehatehate those commercials.

I understand that there are many women who feel less than attractive or lonely because they are fat.

I commend those that take steps to feel better.

But, I don't agree with the fact that the only way to be happy is to be thin.

(I say that over and over because I want people to realize that not all problems are solved by being thin.)

I know that it is a business for these companies. Their goal is to make money so they play on insecurities to get you to look at yourself and say "I am lonely. I am miserable. I need to lose weight to solve the problems."

I would like for you, while reading this handbook, to really think about what it is that will make you truly happy.
If it's joining Jenny Craig or Weight Watchers or just deciding to be happy as you are and eat a little healthier, make **YOURSELF** happy.

That's all that counts.

Let's do this...

First of all, take a good look at the word FAT and the effect it has had on our lives. Many of us remember hearing the word since forever. Many of us can't forget the first time we heard it and had our feelings hurt by it. I was ALWAYS called fat. There is no specific moment in time for me. It's just something I've always heard. One thing can be agreed upon though: It always has the same hurtful effect. No matter if we were little kids, teenagers or adults. It hurts. I tried my best throughout my school years to try and fit in as much as could. I never wanted attention drawn to myself. I knew I was different and we all know that "different" when you're in school means "freak" or "weirdo". I recall how I felt as if it happened yesterday. That is something that never leaves you. But at what point do you realize that FAT is just a word? Who knows? Probably when you reached adulthood and you realized that the world and the people in it are crazy and screwed up. Or maybe even when you realized that words only have power if you let them get to you. Every time you hear it, it puts another dent in your human emotional armor. Doesn't it? Lord knows I have hundreds of chinks and dents in my armor. But you know what? Everyday that I wake up, it still manages to shine. I have finally stopped being hurt by the word. That's why I say it with such ease.

Fat. Haha. Learn to laugh at it or you'll never get past the hurt of it all.

I've learned to tell people that fat is something that can be considered as temporary. But ugly is something that can't be changed. Not even with plastic surgery.

So what if I'm fat? I have to live in this skin, not anyone else. I'm not saying that I couldn't stand to shed some poundage, but, if I don't, my world will not end. Neither will yours. Besides, I happen to enjoy food. I like tasting and sampling different things. I like doing it without the constant thought of "Oh my God, this brownie will put an extra half of a half of a pound on my hips". WHO CARES!!! Eat the damn brownie already!!!

Stop letting some fool tell you that you're not good enough, will never be good enough, if you don't lose weight-change yourself-look like someone else. It's ok to be comfortable being any way that YOU want to be. Whether you want to lose weight or have gotten comfortable with the fat rolls that nest comfortably on your sides. It is up to you. I for one know that I will never be small. I will always be a big girl whether or not I lose weight. And that is fine by me.

Fat folks don't worry about gaining weight. It's already there for goodness sakes! I for one will not worry about the extra pounds while I enjoy my Oreo cookies. Matter of fact, could you pass me another one please?

Now, I talked but the addictions that people have to food that make them gain weight. It's no different from a person who binges and purges to have a small body. It is a disorder. Plain and simple. But, it is not everyone's reason for being fat. Sometimes, you just get comfortable that way.

I have taken it upon myself to try and get people to change their thinking when it comes to fat people. Why, do you ask am I turning this into my own crusade? Honestly? I have no earthly idea. It is an almost impossible task in a world where perfect beauty and thin bodies rule. I guess I have finally gotten tired of being told that I am not good enough-pretty enough-thin enough to even be happy in MY OWN SKIN.
How dare they.
I am me.
Simply put.

There is something else that I wonder about as well.

Why are there books for LIFE IMPROVEMENT, 30 DAY DIET, HOW TO LIVE A STRESS FREE LIFE AND LOSE WEIGHT AT THE SAME TIME IN 10 DAYS, SELF HELP-SELF MEDICATE-UNHAPPY SELF CHANGE YOUR LIFE SELF CHANGE YOUR BODY SELF HELP improvement books EVERYWHERE. But what about books for people who are happy being THEMSELVES. Whether they are fat or not. Where is that section in the bookstore?

Oh wait, I just found it.

In the non-existent section.

Why must everyone on earth insist that people cannot be happy being fat? And when did it become such a crime to be fat.

Arrest this woman, she's overweight.

Who cares.

Really.

I know it isn't easy being different from everyone else, it takes a lot of courage to stand out from the crowd. But is it really that serious? I mean, this FEAR OF FATNESS as I affectionately call it, has gotten out of control. It has turned into a very serious situation. When a woman who is 5'6 and 130 pounds thinks she's fat because some guy said she had a roll of skin on her back starts to think about getting plastic surgery, then yes, it's uncontrollable. People are scared of fatness. Hell, people are scared of chubbiness for that matter. People are scared of anything that gives a little indication that fatness may be on the way.

And it's so sad. Someone will get praise and applause because they decided to have some kind of surgery to lose weight or to change their appearance. I think that is all so very wonderful when people can do things that help them to feel better. But what about those folks who say 'Hey, I'm happy being fat and looking this way. I don't think there's anything wrong with it.'

Oh my lord. Did she just say she's happy being a big fat cow? That's impossible.

Yeah, I said it, so what?

Suddenly people get quiet when you announce to them you're happy just the way you are instead of crying about how much you hate your body and yourself. People seem almost offended when you say things like that. They give you a look like you just shot them in the foot or something.

What's wrong with people who are happy being just the way they are?

Let me give all of you a little insight here:
Being fat isn't easy. Every fat person in the world knows that. But does it mean you aren't human because you're fat? Does it mean that you are doomed to a life of unhealthiness and laziness? Does it mean that (gasp) you are some poor pitiful soul that the fit people look upon and say "He/She is a walking social casualty"?

No.
It doesn't.

You want to know what people think when they see a fat person?

Here you go, a little peek into the "thin" person's mind when it comes to fat folks:

"Fat women always have a misconception on men, and why men over-look fatties for "gym bunnies." It is not so much an issue of attractive (of course there is that, fat is pretty yuck) but more importantly, and always overlooked by the fat ones is that being fat is a direct indicator of a total lack of will power and/or selfish gluttony. Fat women are women who refuse to exercise and eat properly. There is no such thing as "born fat" or "fat gene" or "big boned." Everyone has a similar skel-etal structure. Being fat is an outward sign of a severe personality prob-lem."
Yeah. And every thin person has a tight grip on their emotional prob-lems.

Here's more:

Dear fat slobs,

You are fat because you choose to be. You do not stop eating because you are worthless selfish slobs, always eating, always eating.

You are disgusting because you choose to waste your life, never exercis-ing, always eating, always eating, always eating.

If I happen to stop by the store on the way back from the gym, GET OUT OF MY WAY so I can get through the snack aisle, hippo.
And this one happens to be my favorite:
Oh my god you obese bastards PLEASE STOP EATING

I almost wretch when I have to WALK IN THE STREET because some camel toe fat machine is taking up THE ENTIRE SIDEWALK

1. Get out of my way
2. Stop eating
3. Don't look at me
4. Kill yourself
5 Thanks

How is that for social acceptance, huh?
It's nice to know what people actually think when they can post their thoughts in anonymous places.

It hurts, doesn't it? Knowing the ugliness that people hold on the inside when they see a fat person coming their way. It affects me and I'm almost 30. But, they're only words and we need to learn how to rise above these negative thoughts. We need to stop letting them get to us, overshadowing who we are. Just because you're fat does not mean you're worthless. I can't stress that enough. I have felt so weak and lost and **worthless** sometimes simply because I am not someone else's standard of what beauty is. You have glimpsed how other people feel, now let's bring out some of the things we feel about our selves:

Worthless
Stupid
Disgusting

Shall I go on? Or are you getting the idea?

We need to stop burying ourselves under all of this negative energy. It's like we are in a coffin and someone keeps shoveling dirt on top of us no matter how much we scream to get out, no one hears us. Stop it. Right now. Let's break out of that coffin and start digging our way out of the hellish pits that we put ourselves in.

The Quest

I've titled this section in such a manner because I am on a search for something. As are the ones who will read this book. Be it happiness, health, acceptance, I don't know just yet. But, I do know this: your inner self needs to be healed before your outside self can be healed. Many of us have experienced the most difficult of situations. And I can relate very easily to most of them. But, you need to ask yourself the most important question: Why have I allowed myself to get this way? Whether it's because you're obese, fat, overweight, anorexic, bulimic, or whatever other dysfunction we may have. We refuse to face the truthful answer that we know is buried under all the pain and denial.

Diet pills, diet plans, diet dos and don'ts won't change the true fact that many are hiding behind the layers. It is a matter of protection. My main statement to my unconscious self was "if I protect my outside with this layer, then my inside, my feelings, won't get hurt." So you feed it. And it grows. It becomes an entity within and of itself.

You know what?
That never works.
The pain is still there.
You just cover it up more and more.

Like I said, we bury ourselves.

Too many of us allow our true beings to be buried underneath all of the human waste and negativity that we grow up with. We spend countless years trying to find satisfaction in losing weight and getting thin and buying smaller clothes. I have spent years trying to drop my excess weight. (Both emotional and physical weight). I've tried just about every pill, diet plan, diet group, and I even went to some over-eaters anonymous meetings…(I went to Shoney's buffet afterwards). That shows just how committed I was to that.

I have been cheating myself all of these years. But now I am headed in the right direction. A direction that will lead me to better health, physically and emotionally. I may always be considered fat by most people's standards, but at least I will be in a better place. And you know what? I can accept that. The transition that needs to take place in order to put all of the pieces together again has to involve 4 points: mind, spirit, body and emotional well being.

Without connecting those points, it can be like building a box without sides. Everything will just fall all over the place. And we don't want that to happen.

So, this is where we meet the "truth train".
Climb on board.

Here it comes, speeding down the tracks, what's on it?

Do you know?

All of those old feelings of never being good enough, feeling used, abused, and just a general feeling of worthlessness is on that train with you. It's packed so tightly, there is no room for the really good luggage.

So, basically, that means you're on this trip without clean underwear.

Your mother would be very upset.

All I'm asking is that we step into the conductor's spot and take some control. The train is headed towards a bridge that hasn't been completed yet. It won't be very pretty if you crash.

Especially if you're not wearing clean underwear.

Mind

Try to remember all of those negative remarks people made to you or about you over the last ten years of your life. How many pages could you fill with those negative words? I'm sure we could all fill the pages of this book and then some.

I know I could.

The first lesson we all need to learn is how to throw away that mental notebook that keeps track of those terrible words that we've heard. We internalize and therefore become what we hear. Negative words, just as positive ones, have a profound effect on us. Maybe more so than the positive words. And I don't care how strong you think you are, those negative words come back to us quicker than the positive ones do.

Here's a story for you:

I can recall being in high school and trying out for the cheerleading squad. I was heavier than the girls on the team, of course, and I knew that because of that I would never make it onto the team. But they couldn't stop me from trying. I practiced every move, every kick, every split, until I had it down. I went in front of those girls that day and gave it my all. Even though I knew they would say I was too fat to be a cheerleader. I just wanted to show them that their words and reactions wouldn't stop me. I got so many compliments on my performance and it made me proud. I walked out of that gym feeling like a million bucks. And it was an incredible feeling. It felt good to put aside all of the negative words that I knew I would hear, all of the words that I had been hearing, just to show those girls that I could do it no matter what. But, I wonder, even now, what happened to my resilient attitude that I had for a few brief moments in time.

It came from inside of me. In my mind. They say "mind over matter" is so important. And it is. Such simplicity shouldn't be hard to find, right?

Wrong.

We've all had our "million dollar" moments in life. We just have to find them and bring them into the present with us. When we tell ourselves that **we** are what's important, it will stick. Look in the mirror and say it or write notes to yourself. Whatever works. But do it. I also suggest reading. It does not matter what you read. Just read something inspiring and inspirational. As long as you occupy your mind with something more than thoughts of food or negative feelings. Reorganizing the junk filled attics that we call our mind is the first, and therefore, the most important step. Writing is a mind strengthening exercise as well. Write down your feelings for the day, keep a diary, or start writing your life story.

Just as long as you keep your mind focused and constantly changing and developing.

I also recommend taking a class or two. You're never too old or young to learn something new. Pick up some of those old hobbies that you dropped years ago. Crafting, sewing, and any other activity that you may have dropped when someone else's negativity became your own. Don't have a hobby? Then get one. It's easy. Just know this: you are not alone anymore. We are all connected and going through this together. Never giving up is the key. Exercising our minds gives us the chance to put the other corners of the box together. And when done properly, the contents stay nice and neat on the inside.

<u>Body</u>

I should be the last person on earth trying to tell someone else how and when to exercise. I'm the epitome of exercise excuses.

"I can't exercise today because my back hurts"

"I can't exercise today because it's raining"

"I can't exercise today! I'm watching Oprah."

You get the idea of it all. We all have our own agendas when it comes to making up excuses. Maybe we're afraid of looking foolish while we do jumping jacks or we're afraid we'll pass some offensive gas while doing sit ups. No matter, though. How many people do you know that actually look good doing sit ups while trying to keep themselves from farting?

No body. Trust me.

I have come to terms with the fact that I will never look good doing exercises. I need to sweat and work hard in order to burn calories. I breathe so hard sometimes; I look like a snorting bull. But, I'm in the privacy of my home with only my kids looking at me and laughing.

"Ha ha…look at mommy's stomach jiggle!"

"Gee mom, I've never seen you turn that color before."

The point of all of this is that no matter where you are, just get up and move around. Exercise isn't the intolerable hell that we think it is. It can be fun. Really.

I know other big people will probably laugh, but it's true. I've learned that even the simplest of things can count for something. Now, I don't do running or swimming. But I love walking and I love dancing. I'll put something in the cd player and call my kids into the room and we all dance and act silly.

There is no joy in the world like laughing with your kids.

Don't you want to be around for them?

That is what the basic question comes down to. Either let the world go on without you or get out into the world and go on with it. I had to examine certain things in my life and change them.
Seriously change them.

I have sat on the sofa in front of the television stuffing myself so much that I couldn't catch my breath. I wasn't getting any exercise.
I did, however, invest in some exercise videos.

Yeah.

I'd spend about 5 minutes doing those things. How sad is that?
But, through it all, I have learned a few things:

1. Richard Simmons is much less annoying than everyone thinks he is. Listening to and watching his workout videos are actually very motivating because they have people of all sizes with him. They have been where we are.

2. Walking gives you the chance to take in nature and other things that you don't notice when you're driving by in a car.

3. You need to push yourself. Stop giving up so easily and do what you know you must do.

I never push myself to the point of extreme pain, but I do push myself to the point where I am very proud of my workout at the end.

In order for our minds to stay healthy, our bodies must follow. Even the smallest bit of exercise can count for something. But don't give up and don't stop there. If you can only do three days of exercise per week for only ten minutes a day, don't be pissed with yourself.

Be proud. And keep going because eventually, you'll be doing more and more without even realizing it. Involve the kids. It's quality time spent with them and the laughter gives you an extra burst of needed energy. The weight will start coming off; your eating habits will change because you feel good about changing your life. You'll also become more focused on your final goal:

Improving your life's' quality.

So, just get up and get moving. Life is what happens while you're sitting on the sofa eating Ben and Jerry's ice cream.

Life is what happens

Life is what happens...

While I sit around eating pint after pint of double chocolate ice cream.

While I drown my dreams in a plateful of french fries.

While my kids grow up without me.

While I keep repeating "one of these days..." that never seems to come.

While I hide under the real me under the layers.

While the world goes on.

And life changes and I stay the same.

~KMD

Stop giving up on yourself and stop giving up on life. You must learn to have faith in yourself even when everyone else's' faith fails you. I know that as long as we keep hiding from the world, one day we'll open our eyes and everything, as we know it will be different.

Embrace change.
Welcome the process.

And get up.

<u>Spirit</u>

This type of issue might be tricky for some folks. When I talk about focusing on your spiritual side, I don't necessarily mean finding a new religion or even picking up on the old one. I am a firm believer in the fact that one can have a personal relationship with God and the universe on one's own terms and in one's own time. Too many people lose the connection between body and spirit when they try to change their lives. There is a certain order that things need to take in order to work properly. Body and spirit actually need to be one with each other, but for the purpose of my book, I split the two. How can you connect exercise and prayer might you ask?

Very easily.

Pray for strength while working out.
Pray for the will to keep going on when you feel like stopping and you know you shouldn't.
Spirit takes over when the body feels like shutting down.
Your physical body can only do so much for itself on its own. The extra push that you get comes from a higher power all around us and within us.
Ever utter the words "how did I ever do that?" after completing something that normally seemed out of your reach?
That's "spiritual intervention". Our spirit knows when to kick in. That higher power that we rely on makes it so.

So, just as you eat to keep your inner body strong and exercise to keep your physical form healthy, so must you tend to your spirit. Feeding it with prayer, meditation, awareness of the world's beauty and a love for self and others. I find that reading daily prayers and meditations keeps me focused on my goal and help to keep me in a positive state of mind and spirit. When you feel better inside, it shows on the outside. Start out however you wish. Just so long as you remember that you need all four sides to keep your box strong.

No one aspect is more important than the other, they all are of equal value.

<u>Daily Mantra</u>

Healing mind heals body.
Healing spirit heals emotions.

Emotional Well Being

Here is my favorite part.
One we can all share war stories about: emotional wear and tear and eventual break down.

I've been there on several occasions.
As I said before, we take all the negative things people say about us and internalize it. We turn ourselves into emotional punching bags for other people who are unhappy with themselves. The key, I suppose, to really getting away from this type of abuse, is to reinforce our own positive opinions of ourselves.

Easier said than done though.

It only takes negative words a moment to break someone down. But it takes months, even years, to build up a positive center of self. One would think that the opposite would be true instead.
What is it about negative words that act so quickly, so brutally, that can ruin ones day or even life.
Let's first examine the power of words themselves. Look at the following list of words and really think about what place they have in your life right now:

joy
depression
laughter
over-eating
stupid
intelligent
fat
beautiful
glutton

Which words jumped out at you?

Probably the ones that you've been hearing on a regular basis.
My guess is, the negative ones are heard more often.

My theory on negative words goes like this: they tear at the layers of our positive self-image. We all have a positive image of ourselves at one point or another. It's almost like peeling an orange. You can't peel the skin off all at once, but piece by piece. Once you have the skin removed, you can rip that orange right in half if you like. Then, you can break it into smaller pieces. The positive words are the pulp of the orange. They hang on for dear life to stay together, but it's impossible when you have such a heavy force pulling at it. That's how negative words work. Positive words have a hard time hanging on. No one ever bothers to say to themselves "hey, who cares what they say…I like myself" on a daily basis. But, we tell ourselves everyday how fat and unhappy we are, how miserable we are…you get the idea. Those tiny pieces of pulp die off when they are separated from the rest of the orange.

So, how much positive reinforcement do you give yourself?

I know I don't do such a good job of it. So I can imagine how many others reading this are just like me.

The first thing in taking a step towards emotional healing and well being is stop letting other people peel our skin away. Even if all you ever hear is negative words, it only takes a moment to say to yourself "I'm a good, beautiful, spiritual person. There is a higher power that thought enough of me to create me. It is now my job to do the rest."

You don't expect half wrapped presents at Christmas do you?

I didn't think so…

So why do a half assed job when it comes to our emotional well being?

We don't give ourselves enough credit to know that we are better than those negative words and negative people. That needs to stop right now. Say out loud that you are going to start at this very moment, taking care of yourself.

So what if you're fat. Are you happy that way? If you are, great!!! Don't let anyone tell you any differently.

If you're not happy being fat, do something about it. But only because you want to. Not because some idiot is telling you that you need to lose weight.

There is a very simple exercise that I would like everyone to perform. Get out a sheet of paper and pen and make two columns. One column is good, the other, bad. List all of those negative feelings and words. Write down all those positive feelings.

Which list is longer?

I've gotten tired of feeling those feelings and hearing those negative words. But I made up my mind that no matter what, I would believe in myself.

Look in the mirror.

Who do you see?

Do you like that person looking back at you?

It doesn't matter if your mother or your sister or your friend or that guy you have a crush on said they don't like the way you are. Do you like yourself?

That is the question of the day.
Maybe even the year.

I bet the person looking back from that reflection is that scared kid who got teased in school and at home for being heavy. The one who was always afraid that no one would like them. That kid is hurt. And they never got the chance to heal.

Give yourself a fair chance and take a real look at how things really are. Life is not easy. But, I can assure you that it's a lot easier when you're in touch with yourself and your emotions.

My Personal Journal

In a way, this book is my journal. It helps me while helping others, to explore those deep-set feelings in my life. I it also helps to keep a journal to record activity, the types of food you eat, when, what type of mood you were in when you ate them and any positive reinforcements. A journal will get you to thinking about things in your everyday life that you never pay attention to. You see, when you write, it gives you the chance to pick apart and examine every feeling, every thought, and every word. When one is going through a "rebirth", whether it is physical, emotional or spiritual, you need to know exactly, and in what detail, the things that need to be changed. Myself, for instance, being a single mom and trying to focus on my goals, put lots of stress in my life. It may not seem that way to those who know me, but, at night when I would try to rest, sleep did not come easily. My mind and my emotions were going at a thousand miles a minute. Things around me were all upset and I couldn't focus. We all have stresses of different types and on different levels going on in our lives. We put up brave faces for the world and pretend that everything is okay. The same thing applies when we talk about weight issues. You may be out in public in front of everyone pretending, faking the fact that you are comfortable in your own skin when the truth is, you're not.

It's time to start focusing and realizing that life as we know it is changing and we need to change with it. This, all of my words and feelings pouring out into these pages, that is what is keeping me focused. It's helped me to face my depression and my weight issues.

If only one person reads this book and it helps them, I will be completely satisfied.

It's all about well-being.

Complete and total well-being.

So, just take a moment to think: is it a weight issue or is it a **_me_** issue?

What is it that makes **_me_** unhappy about…(apply your own situations here)

Are you unhappy because you're fat or are you unhappy because other people don't like the fact that you're fat?

Have you taken on their opinion of you and turned it into your opinion of yourself?

Or is it because you think no one will like you because you're fat?

I know there are people out there who give these amazing speeches and have extraordinary stories about how much their lives have changed since they lost weight. They are very moving and inspirational things to hear. It does get you to thinking about losing weight and making an improvement in your life.

You say "wow, that's great. Maybe if I get on track and eat better and exercise I will improve my life as well."

But is weight your real issue? That is what you need to think about before getting all gung-ho and jumping up on the bandwagon.

Will you be more or less satisfied once the weight is gone?

I have to ask myself the same questions.
As easy to answer as they may sound, these are very difficult questions to answer. Using myself as an example, I sometimes go from wanting to lose weight to not wanting to lose because I get comfortable with myself sometimes. So, switching yourself from one pole to the other isn't the best thing. Your decision has to be a definitive one.
Either you are or you aren't.
I have made the connection after years of emotional issues, weight issues and life issues.
I like me.

Just as I am.

But I also know that carrying too much extra weight is a potential danger to my health.

I needed to start from the inside out to make the connection to even begin to decide about making a change. We all need to start seeing ourselves in a better, brighter light. It's not an easy journey, but, know this, there are many, many others out there taking the journey with you.

<u>Daily Mantra</u>

"Either do not attempt it at all
Or
Go through with it."
~OVID

The Time Is Now

Time seems to stand still sometimes in a fat person's life. I know more often than not in my own life: missed opportunities and chances. Plenty of missed things. But I will not let it continue that way. Life should be a joyride. Not a nightmare with some blind crazy person sitting behind the wheel.

At what point did you let go of the steering wheel?

I can only reflect on all the things I have missed out on because I let myself become down right miserable.

My kids
My family
MY LIFE

Who wants to continue to miss out on things like that?
Not me.
And you shouldn't want to either.

Look back at all the things that have come and gone in your life while you sat around being unhappy. Now look forward and promise yourself that life will never get away from you again. And although life certainly has a way with testing our determination and our resolve, you can get through **_anything_** that comes your way.
This isn't a "how I changed my life in five simple steps" thing. This is about taking time to change and for all the right reasons.

But of course, we all wish it could be changed in five simple steps.

Just give yourself an honest shot at moving forward and I can promise you that you'll feel better in no time. And although the rent is cheap in the emotional dumping ground that we tend to live, it's better on the side of emotional wellness. Plus you get a big back yard free of all the trash.

Have you seen me?
I'm not sure where the ME I once knew went

Has anyone seen ME?
I think ME got lost somewhere between social acceptance and society's standard

I wish I knew where ME was

Are you sure you've never, ever seen ME?
How I wish you had

ME was so wonderful and bright and funny
But foolishly I dropped ME, somewhere

Just thinking about ME makes my heart ache
I know ME is lonely

ME made I feel accepted
But without ME, I am nothing

So, just in case you see ME, tell ME that I am searching
I will never give up
I will search forever
And I will never give ME up again

~KMD

The Real Deal

I can go on and on about weight issues and emotional issues and any other issues that may exist. But I won't do that because I feel as though the people that hold this book in their hands already know what it's like to face the same issues over and over again. What we should face is the fact that we are self-destructive. God gave us bodies to take care of and we destroy it with all of our addictions. That person we face in the mirror everyday isn't the real person that lies deep with in us. We need to see with our hearts and our minds in order to find the person that hides beneath it all. Yes. We wish we had firm butts, perky breasts and flat stomachs. But life isn't perfect. By any stretch of the imagination. And truth be told, we do wish sometimes that we looked like those perfect people on television. I often find myself admiring the perfectly chiseled bodies of the women on television: videos, celebrities, models. It makes me wonder about my own body and how abnormal or hideous every seems to think it is. I also find myself wondering "If I looked like that, how different would my life be."

Well, I will never look like the girls on television. Or like the girls that grace pages of magazines. It does make me envious at times, but I am me and I need to learn to live with that.

You can't have a positive attitude all the time, I admit that.

There are times when it will all get you so down that you won't be able to stand it. But, you also need to learn how to love and accept yourself the way you are now. Then you can move on and maybe stay at a positive place in your life. Besides, if you do work hard enough and end up looking somewhere near to what the models and video girls look like, that doesn't mean you'll be happy, either.

You want to know what my biggest disappointment is in this whole situation?

The fashion industry.

I feel like just because we are fat, they abandon us. Yes, I know they make clothes in our sizes, but have you seen some of the models they put these things on? I mean really. Look at some of the catalogs. I know I'm not the only one that has noticed.

A woman who wears a size 6 wearing a flowered lounge dress in a catalog advertising up to a size 44?

Yeah, that makes sense. She's just dying to lounge around in a fat woman's moomoo.

I know when I am catalog shopping I say to myself "gee, I wonder what that would like in a size 10 even though I am in a size 28."

Come on now.

I'm a big girl. And big girls want to see other big girls modeling clothes. I want to see someone that resembles **_me_**. I want to see a gal with fat arms wearing a sleeveless dress. Not some skinny woman with skinny arms. My arms don't look like that. I want to know what those clothes will look like on me. Why not make advertising more appealing to the women you cater to? Why make them feel even worse about themselves by using models that don't even fit in any of the clothes? We are ignored by the fashion industry. They sometimes design things that hide our beauty rather than actually show it off.
I wouldn't cover my car with some of the things they make.

We just need to be more vocal about our fashions.
Stand up and tell the fashion industry that fat girls can be sexy too.

Another thing that has come to light is that 130-pound women are being considered "full figured"?!

What?

The other day, my girlfriend and I were standing at the checkout at a store and we were thumbing through some magazines. The pages were filled with pictures of different stars and the caption reads "they are not afraid to have curves on their 130 full figures." We screamed with laughter. And then the thought settled in.

They don't know what it's really like to be considered "full figured" or "plus sized". They have never had to deal with rejection because they were too heavy. They don't know what it's like to hate yourself because everyone thinks you're some kind of freak.

They don't what it's like to struggle with being fat and praying for acceptance.

Ii resent that they even think they come close to being "full figured".

And I hate the fact that the world today tells fat people they should hate themselves for being fat.

And I hate the fact that I let them make me feel that way.

I look at women everyday, all types of women, complaining that they hate their bodies because of an extra 10 pounds that no one else seems to notice. and even when you tell them they are beautiful, they still aren't satisfied.

Doomed to forever hating and changing themselves.

When will people realize that looks aren't everything.

Maybe never.

But what can you do, as a woman especially, when any and everything in the world revolves around what you look like and how much you weigh. You can do nothing, I guess, but either go crazy, adapt to it or live on the outskirts of acceptance.

In a place that says they welcome and celebrate differences, being different makes you unacceptable.

And did I miss the meeting that the world had about everybody looking like everybody else?
Look at all the singers. Suddenly, everybody's blonde.

The world will be forever locked in a battle to look "good".
People will never be satisfied being blonde, thin or whatever.
People should learn to be happy being themselves no matter how imperfect we may be. Differences are what make us interesting.

And you know what?

I think I kinda like being different.

Do I want to fit in or do I want to fit out?
It's hard sometimes figuring this shit out

Everyone wants "attractive and athletic"
Well, I'm not either, so I guess I'm just pathetic

Why do I let these thoughts slip into my mind?
Making me hate myself, it's so unkind

Whatever happened to looking for "sincere and witty"?
I guess it's been replaced by the butt implant and
the fake titty

I guess I'm just a social casualty,
Existing on the brink of insanity

Where did "I want someone nice" go?
Oh, yeah, it's been replaced by "I want a woman who's
a ho"

Is it too much to dream of finding someone who wants
to love me
for being comfortable with me being the best me I can
be

That is what I want everyone to see,
I'm just ME

Simple and plain,
somewhere close to being sane

Is it too much to ask?
It can't be that impossible of a task

I know he is out there and he's looking to share his
Life
and make a girl like me his wife

He doesn't know me yet
but with me, happiness is what he'll get

So keep on looking my dear,
I'll be waiting right here

Relationships

How many times have you found yourself in a so-called "relationship" with someone just because you felt like you couldn't do better?

I know I have been in that type of situation more than I care to remember. Or more than I care to admit, I should say.

I think fat people in general feel this need to be connected to others in a specific way simply because it makes us feel more accepted.
In wanting to feel accepted, we reject those parts of ourselves that constantly tell us we deserve better.

We ignore our senses.

We ignore everything that tells us that the person we are dealing with is treating us like crap. All because we want to be able to say "I'm in a relationship with someone."

Too often we don't put enough value on ourselves. We feel as though we are not worthy of the love, respect, the **SELF RESPECT** that we should be giving ourselves instead of depending on some asshole to give it to us. Just because we are fat doesn't mean that we are not worthy.

I think that sentence bears repeating:

<u>JUST BECAUSE WE ARE FAT DOES NOT MEAN THAT WE ARE NOT WORTHY OF LOVE AND RESPECT</u>.

But more important than any other relationship is the one we have ***WITH OURSELVES***.

Why do we continue to put up with being used and mistreated anyway?

Is it the self-hate that we feel that makes us do this? Or is it the hate that we have for the people who hate fat people?

I don't know what category I would fall into with this one because I have had many, many relationships where I have been used or abused emotionally. And it is no one else's fault but my own because I let myself fall victim to those that prey upon women with low self esteem. They can pick us out in a crowd because they think "She's fat. She hates herself."

And most of the time, they are correct with that line of thinking.

But, I shouldn't just put women into that "easy prey" category because it happens to fat men as well. Women pick them out just as easily and crush their emotional well-being.

I guess I need to be as honest as possible here and let you all know more about my sordid past.
It's a long story but I am more than willing to share it all…

I can't exactly say when I lost my sense of self and started giving into the weaknesses that eventually consumed the better part of me. I'm sure you can understand when I say that my need for companionship was greater than my need for self-respect. I once dated a guy that in one breath would say he loved me and in the next say he thought I was too fat and that I would look better if I dropped some weight.

Yes. I was desperate.

Why? He wasn't even all that great. He had emotional problems and other issues that didn't exactly make him the best catch. For me or any-one else for that matter. But, I tolerated him, his problems, and his insults. It was the most degrading thing ever and after he was through with me I felt like I had been dumped in a landfill. My **SELF** was ruined. Not forever mind you, but it was damaged pretty badly. I still feel the effects of his awfulness.

So, I am not just speaking on something that I have no experience with. I can tell more stories, but the details are too sordid to put onto these pages.
But, I know where you are and I know where you've been.
I know the pit that being used puts you into.

I'm also here to let you know that you can climb out of it.

It's not easy letting go of yourself to give it to another person who only uses it and crushes it in the blink of an eye. We ignore so many things because we want to feel the closeness, the acceptance that someone else expresses to us. But, when it turns out to be just a game to them, the damage is sometimes irreversible.

Fat folks should stop letting themselves be easy prey for the vultures that get off from using us to get themselves to the next level.

You know the type I'm talking about. The guys that use fat chicks for easy sex. Or money. Or a place to stay. Whatever you have to offer them at that point in time.

Yeah, you say?

Still in that spot aren't you?

Well, get the fuck out of it. Because you know what? The next pretty, thin blonde that comes through, he'll dump you quicker than you can say "Jenny Craig".

And how will that make you feel?

Like shit right?

The same way you've so many times before.

And that's not right.

You're not being fair to yourself or to the guy that will come along and love you just as you are: Fat and beautiful.

Yes.

Fat and beautiful.

(So, don't give him a hard time when he comes along because you stuck with the loser guy and he messed over you.)

So let's get down to the basics of what it's all about as women, shall we?...

I won't apologize for being so graphic in this section because I am telling the truth and speaking on something that I know so much about. And what does it all come down to anyway?
Being desired **SEXUALLY.**

That is the ultimate thing that can make or break a relationship. (Don't agree, but it's a proven fact)

A guy "falls in love" with you or likes you simply because of how you look instead of getting to know about you and who you are. Suddenly, you get comfortable and start packing on the pounds and he doesn't love you anymore.
You're still the same person, just not a size 8 anymore.
But still he deserts you.

That means he didn't really appreciate or love you for the PERSON that is beneath the sexy body and tight clothes.
What happens when you're 75 and your ass is sagging and your boobs are touching your knees? Will he not love you anymore at that point in life?

The point I'm trying to make is this: Love me now as I am, for what I might become, and when I'm a saggy assed old woman.

We all dream of the guy that will come along one day and sweep us off of our feet (not literally). And he does exist. We just need to know when and where he comes along. But, if we spend time being used and abused, then we will become jaded and angry and we'll miss the chance to meet him.

Not only is that loser ruining your self esteem, he's ruining your chances of meeting the real deal guy that will love you and your fat rolls.

I'm trying to wait as patiently as possible for my one and only so I know it takes plenty of strength. But it will happen. Eventually.

I know that I didn't put any value on myself or my feelings for a very long time. But, I don't suppose I should refer to it as something that is in the past. I still do it.

Why?
Like I said, negative thinking/behavior is hard to break.
But just because it's hard to break doesn't mean it can't be broken.

At this point in my life, I am completely single. I can't put that on the fact that I am fat though because even Halle Berry has men troubles.

I am single because I am waiting for my one and only to come along and I don't want to compromise my "I am great the way I am so take it or leave it" attitude.

Yes, I get lonely.

Yes, I get bored.

But, I also know that I am worthy of that one and only true love that has pined for me for so many years just as I have pined for him.

I'm asking that you take yourself into consideration and wait for your one and only.
If we don't respect our feelings and love ourselves first, we certainly can't expect anyone else to do it for us.

So, stand up for yourself and decide today, **RIGHT NOW** that you are worthy of all the happiness in the world.

I HAVE SOME SUGGESTIONS:

Be sure to do things for yourself
Appreciate yourself (No one else will do it for you)
Shop for yourself (My favorite)

Whatever it is, be good to yourself instead of waiting on someone else to be good to you.

I can't stress enough the points about loving and accepting yourself. Once you do that, there is no limit to where you can go in life or what you can do. Have confidence in yourself ALWAYS. Life has so much to offer.

So, go out and live it, be it and **LOVE IT!!!**

TODAY, I WILL BE RESPONSIBLE FOR MY OWN HAPPINESS. I WILL NOT LET THE COMMERCIALS, VIDEOS, MODELS OR SOCIETY DICTATE TO ME WHAT I SHOULD LOOK LIKE IN ORDER TO BE HAPPY.

TODAY, I WILL LOVE ME. I WILL ACCEPT ME THE WAY I AM. I WILL LOVE EVERY FAT ROLL, EVERY CURVE, EVERY CREASE. I WILL LOVE ME JUST AS I AM.

TODAY WILL BE A NEW CHAPTER IN MY LIFE STORY.

SHAME ON YOU FAT GIRL...

I could say I'm a BBW, but why lie?
I'm just a fat girl

I could say I'm Voluptuous, but why lie?
I'm just a fat girl

I could say Robust, Full-Figured, or Big-Boned, but why lie?
I'm just a fat girl

Not accepted in this non-fat, low-fat world,
just a fat girl reject,

But even if you don't like my roundness,
I LOVE MYSELF
And all my fatness

In all my fatty girl glory,

I can say BBW, BIG BONED, CURVACEOUS, VOLUPTUOUS
but why lie?

I'm just a fat assed fat girl...

~KMD

<u>NEON</u>

Flowing through life's existence,
Only to exist

Feeling disconnected,
Lonely and Undiscovered

Should I burn as brightly as the neon in the sky?

Should I?

If only to burn as brightly

Why try?

I still go unnoticed

Still existing to simply exist

I am my own stranger,
Jealous of the neon burning brightly in the sky

Should I?
Should I?

Dare to even try?

~KMD

BE YOUR OWN CHEERLEADER...

With all of the things that I have discussed here, my experiences, my feelings, I am learning so much more about myself than I ever thought possible. It is very hard to come to terms with the fact that sometimes, you are just who you are. And you are **JUST FINE.**

As I sit here writing this, I have my moments of wanting to lose weight and be someone else's "Ideal" woman. But, is that really being true to myself?

No, it isn't.

I know we all fall short somewhere in our lives, but, we should never fall short when it comes to our feelings and our self-image. We are our best, and sometimes only, cheerleaders. And that is perfectly okay.

Now, don't get me wrong, I'm not saying not to exercise and get healthy, I'm just saying that your idea should not be "I need to lose weight in order to be happy". I have said it over and over, **YOU DON'T NEED TO BE THIN IN ORDER TO BE HAPPY.**

That is something we should tell ourselves all the time. Stop being cheated out of life. Do you have any idea how many times people say "When I lose weight I'll do this and that".

You know what? Sometimes, this and that never comes around.

Never.

Remember that next time you put off that cruise or those new clothes or LIFE because you feel as though you're not thin enough.
Life doesn't happen because you're thin, it happens because you live it.

And I should learn to take my own advice. Which is why I'm writing this handbook. (SMILES)

People who know me may be shocked when they read these words because I tend not to share my feelings about being fat with others. Not even those who are very close to me. It's odd that I have no problems sharing these feelings with strangers.

Maybe I should start.

But, you can't just go around telling people "Hey, you're fat but it shouldn't stop you from living."

So, the best way for me to do that is by writing this handbook. This way, I can let hundreds of women know that they are JUST FINE the way they are.

So many will disagree with that statement.
But I really don't give a rat's patootie about it.

HAHAHA.

It feels so good to just say it. **I DON'T CARE WHAT YOU THINK ABOUT ME.**

It is refreshing to start the process of getting out of the chains of other people's opinions.

The only REAL opinion that counts is the opinion we have of ourselves.

We also need to learn that everyone else's opinion about us shouldn't become OUR opinion about ourselves.

Did you all get that?

Your opinion is the only one that counts when it comes to you and living your life the way you choose to live it.

Besides, opinions are like buttholes. Everybody has one.
And sometimes, what comes out, really stinks.

**SOMEONE ELSE'S OPINION OF ME ISN'T THE
OPINION I HAVE OF MYSELF.
LET THEM HAVE THEIR NEGATIVE THOUGHTS.
I WILL NOT LET THEM AFFECT ME ANY LONGER.**

DON'T JUDGE ME

Don't call me cruel names
Just because I'm happy being me

Besides,
Being me is the best way to be

With a swagger in my walk
And happiness in my voice

Don't judge me

Because you try to fit in
With a difficult society

And in case you didn't know,
It's not working for you

Try being you

With a pep in your step
And a smile on your face

Tell it to the world
Say it when you speak

Being me is the best thing to be

Don't judge me

Because I'm me

Twitching my hips
Smiling when I talk

I don't want to hear
"Why does she flaunt all of that?"

Because I'm me
And that's the best way to be

AND ONE MORE TIME FOR EMPHASIS...

In ending this handbook, I want every woman to know that confidence is the key to your success and happiness. Many nights I have suffered and cried because I depended on other peoples' image instead of my own.

Many nights I have looked in the mirror and said how much I have hated and despised my big, fat, round, squishy body.

Many nights I have thought that the only way I would find happiness was to be thin.

Many nights I have wanted to kill myself because I thought being fat was the worst thing in the world.

Like I said before, this handbook has been my therapy, my revelation, my joy and my purpose: IT HAS TAUGHT ME TO LOVE MYSELF. UNCONDITIONALLY. COMPLETELY. And I want it to do the same for you.

Life won't be easy. And we won't always be accepted the way we are. But we also need to make our way in life. Don't expect anyone to respect you the way you are. You need to demand it and show them that fat or not, **I AM HAPPY AND PROUD TO BE A FAT ASSED FAT GIRL...**

~Kimberly M. Denesse, Fat Girl Extraordinaire

THE END

My stomach is squishy and soft,
My ass jiggles when I walk,
My arms flap like turkey wings,
My thighs rub together,

But no one loves me more than I do
Only I can see the beauty in all these rolls and curves

My neck is thick,
My chin is double,

But no one loves me more than I do
Only I can see the beauty in all these rolls and curves

I am me,
Just the way I am,

A fat girl
Round and proud.

~Kimberly M. Denesse

978-0-595-38391-7
0-595-38391-2